Wall Pilates and Chair Exercises for Seniors Over 50

28 Days Easy Low Impact Workouts to Strengthen and Improves Flexibility, Posture and Balance

Giovanni Gonzalez

Disclaimer

Before embarking on any exercise program outlined in this book, it is imperative that you seek guidance from a qualified healthcare professional or an experienced exercise professional. The author and publishers of this book bear no responsibility for any injuries or damages that may occur as a result of applying the information provided.

It is crucial to recognize that each individual is unique, possessing varying levels of physical condition and health. This book is a general guide and may not cater to specific health conditions or individual circumstances. Always listen to your body, refrain from pushing yourself beyond your limits, and modify exercises according to your personal abilities and conditions.

Please be aware that engaging in the exercises suggested in this book involves inherent risks. It is essential to perform them with care, responsibility, and mindfulness of your own capabilities.

Prioritize safety by executing the exercises in an appropriate environment, utilizing stable and suitable equipment.

The information provided in this book is not a substitute for professional medical advice, diagnosis, or treatment. Consult with your physician or a qualified healthcare provider before commencing any exercise program, especially if you have pre-existing health conditions, concerns, or are taking medication.

Copyright © 2023 by Giovanni Gonzalez

The views and opinions expressed in this book are solely those of the author. The author has made every reasonable effort to ensure that the information provided in this book is accurate and up to date at the time of publication.

Table of Contents

PART I: WALL PILATES FOR SENIORS OVER 50

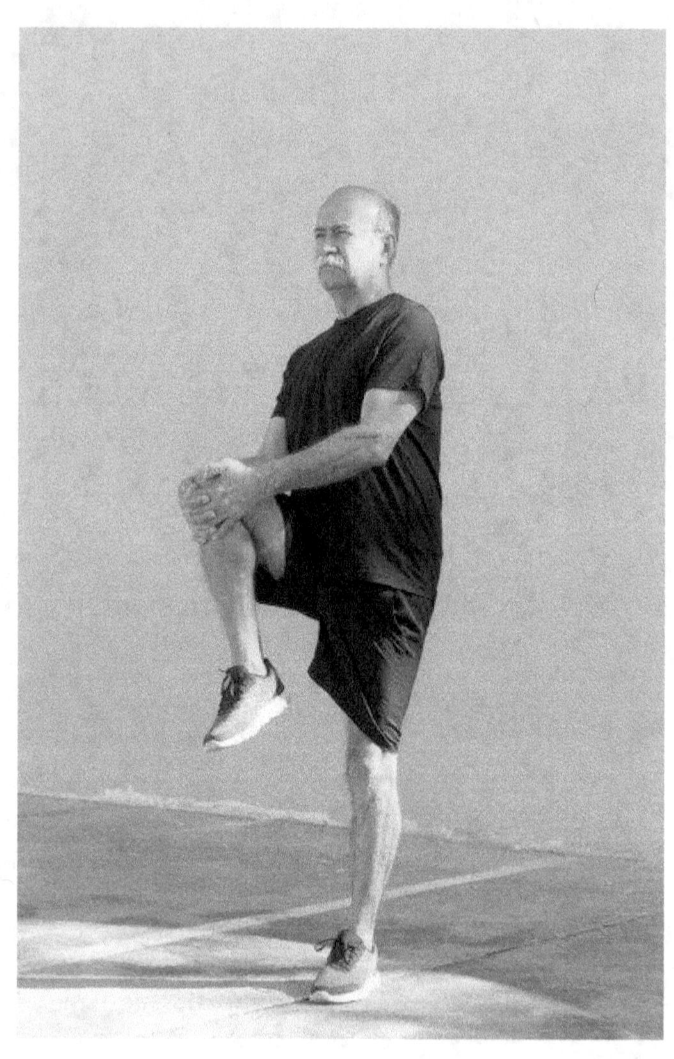

INTRODUCTION

In a world where aging and its relentless march on us can often leave us feeling lethargic and depressed, exercise is a potent remedy that can revitalize not only our physical selves but also our entire existence.

Imagine escaping the bonds of persistent discomfort and aches, saying goodbye to sluggishness, and welcoming a future full of energy and fulfillment. **Wall Pilates for Seniors Over 50** is a simple yet revolutionary technique that holds the key to accessing this tremendous potential.

Introducing Emily, a middle-aged woman who, like many others, became ensnared in the cycle of excessive sedentary lifestyles and poor energy. Her story is similar to many others' until an insightful article about the significant benefits of exercise gave her a breakthrough. It provided the spark she was lacking and offered a glimmer of hope for a future free from the challenges she faced.

Encouraged by the prospect of a better day ahead, Emily bravely decided to start including Wall Pilates in her everyday regimen. The results were nothing short of remarkable in a matter of weeks.

A burst of vitality shot through her veins, dispelling the cloud of exhaustion that had descended upon her. Weight started to drop off, and each session brought her back to her previous level of confidence as well as her physical strength. Emily's experience with Wall Pilates went beyond simple physical fitness and instead opened the door to an amazing trip she had never dared to imagine.

For individuals navigating their senior years, **Wall Pilates for Seniors over 50** offers a beacon of transforming strength in a world when pursuing health and vitality frequently feels like an uphill battle. This is more than just a workout plan; it's a means to an enhanced sense of strength and flexibility that will lead to a comfortable and contented existence.

Imagine a trainer who not only recognizes and honors the potential for strength and resilience that exists within seniors, but also comprehends their specific requirements. Greetings from a seasoned fitness trainer expert writing a thorough journey that aims to redefine the aging experience. The main advantages open up before you like pages in a book as you go through this deep investigation, with every turn exposing possibilities for a revitalized existence.

With its benefits for improved muscle tone and flexibility, wall Pilates acts as a catalyst for both a physical and mental recovery. However, the story doesn't end there; it goes all the way to the very center of you, promising a power that seeps into every aspect of your everyday life.

Wall Pilates for Seniors Over 50 is so beautiful because it may increase your power on all levels—mentally, physically, and emotionally. Imagine doing everyday chores with fresh ease and experiencing a resurgence of energy while taking on activities that you used to find difficult.

I'm your reliable personal trainer guide, your author. I have painstakingly designed activities that will build your body and spirit while inspiring ageless confidence. The activities and knowledge shared in this book is the outcome of years of experimental research, training and experience learned.

This is a guidebook to a life where every movement is met with strength, every obstacle is overcome with perseverance, and every day is welcomed with a feeling of success rather than merely a fitness manual. Come along on this life-changing adventure with us as we explore the world of Wall Pilates.

The book's pages open to reveal not just exercises but also a route to a life full of energy and the delight of discovering new talents. Find out how to reach your full potential and let me lead you to a future in which strength is ageless.

Importance of Exercise for Seniors

The importance of consistent exercise for elders grows as the passing of time elegantly marks life's journey. Being physically active is not only a decision; it is a fundamental aspect of aging well that offers both short-term and long-term advantages.

1. Health and Wellness: Seniors' physical health can be enhanced and maintained with regular exercise. It supports stronger bones and muscles, better cardiovascular health, and weight management. Exercise creates a strong and healthy body by lowering the risk of chronic illnesses and improving balance and flexibility.

2. Cognitive Health: Exercise has benefits for cognitive health in addition to physical health. According to studies, engaging in regular physical activity can help people age with better memory, increased cognitive function, and a lower chance of cognitive decline. Exercise turns into a comprehensive treatment plan for preserving brain clarity and developing mental agility.

3. Emotional Resilience: Exercise also has compelling emotional benefits. Regular physical activity might help seniors feel less stressed, anxious, and depressed. Exercise causes the body's natural mood enhancers, endorphins, to be released, which improves mood and makes you feel good about life.

4. Social Connection: Exercise provides seniors with valuable opportunities for social interaction. Whether through exercise courses, walking groups, or fitness activities, promotes a sense of camaraderie and fights feelings of loneliness. Exercise's social component adds to a happy and connected way of living.

5. Increased Self-Sufficiency: For elders, maintaining their independence is of utmost importance. Maintaining functional independence and mobility requires regular exercise. It gives people the confidence to complete everyday chores, which lessens their need for outside help and increases their sense of independence.

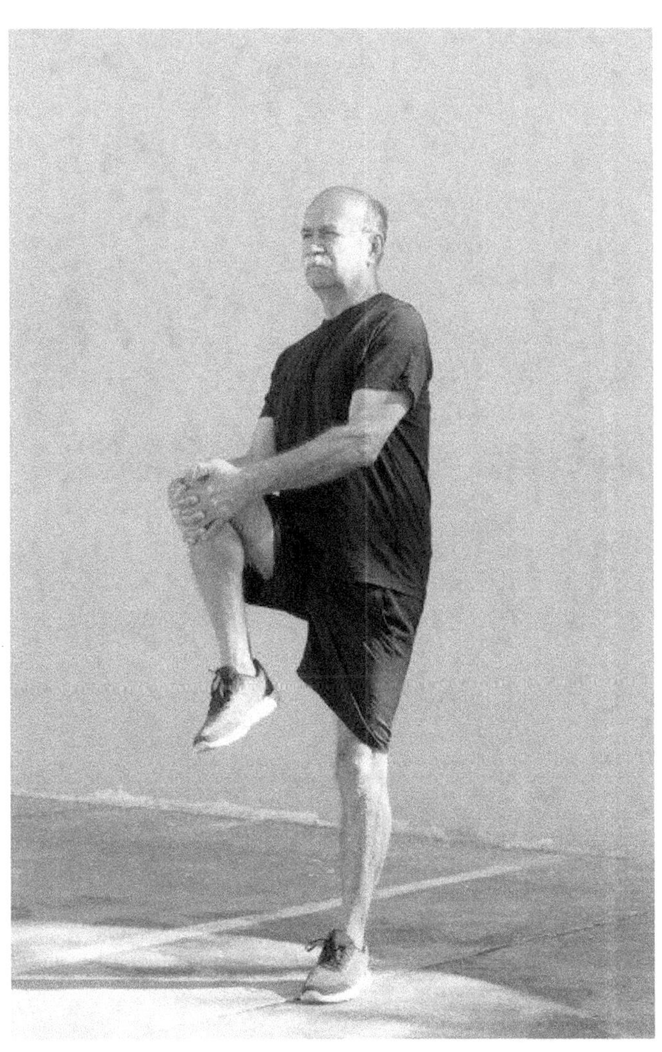

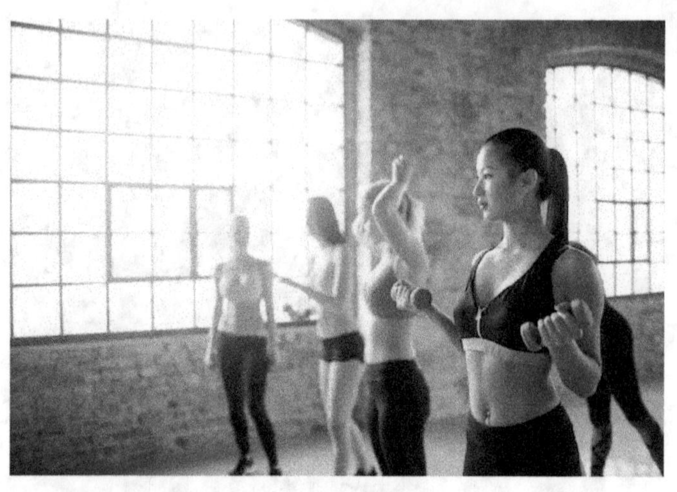

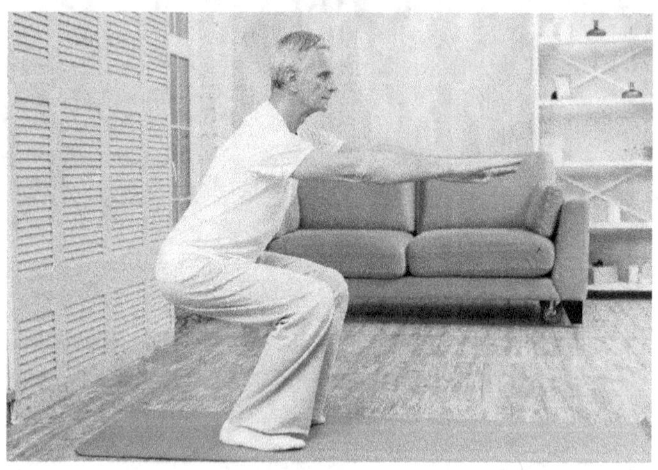

CHAPTER ONE
Understanding Wall Pilates

A specific method to training known as wall Pilates combines the ideas of classical Pilates with the extra element of a wall for support. This combination produces a special, stable atmosphere that is very helpful for seniors who are 50 years of age and older. Focusing on deliberate breathing, controlled movements, and core activation, wall Pilates offers a thorough exercise program that goes beneath the surface to develop strength, flexibility, and balance.

Principle of Wall Pilates

Basic ideas that govern the technique and increase its effectiveness are the core principles of Wall Pilates:

1. Main Engagement: In the center of Wall Pilates involves using your core muscles, which include your lower back, pelvic floor, and abdominals. This fundamental idea promotes stability, enhances posture, and builds total body strength.

2. Breath Awareness: A key component of Wall Pilates, conscious breathing encourages a coordinated relationship between breath and movement. Seniors can become more adept at using their muscles to contract and relax by practicing deliberate breathing in and out.

3. Control and Precision: Wall Pilates emphasizes controlled, exact movements. By practicing intentional movement, participants reduce their chance of strain or injury. This idea guarantees that every exercise helps to specifically strengthen and tone specified muscle areas.

Advantages of Wall Pilates for Seniors

Wall Pilates offers a multitude of benefits for adults over 50 and is also designed to meet their demand. The advantages go beyond gains in physical health and include mental health and an overall improvement in quality of life.

Improved Posture

The obvious posture improvement that comes with Wall Pilates is one of its most notable benefits for seniors. An erect and self-assured stance is encouraged by the emphasis on spinal alignment and core activation. Seniors who engage in certain exercises become more conscious of how their bodies are positioned, which helps them maintain a more poised and graceful gait.

Increased Flexibility

The natural aging process is a common issue for seniors and can cause joint stiffness and decreased flexibility. Wall Pilates incorporates fluid movements and gentle stretches into its program to address these issues. By focusing on certain muscle groups, these workouts help to develop range of motion and flexibility. Seniors move more comfortably and easily throughout everyday tasks as their flexibility increases.

Enhanced Strength

Wall Pilates is an effective way for seniors to develop and preserve their strength. Using the wall as a supporting structure enables the regulated activation of different muscle groups. This type of focused strength training promotes improved stability and resilience in addition to assisting in the fight against the loss of muscle that comes with aging. Seniors who advance through the program gain greater strength, which translates into a stronger and more capable physical state.

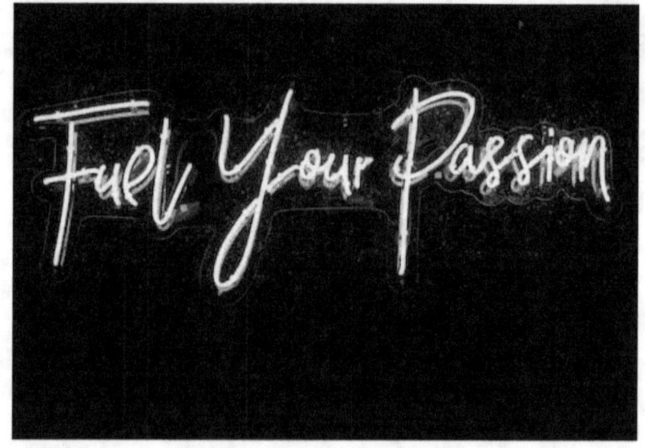

CHAPTER TWO
Getting Started with Wall Pilates

For seniors, starting Wall Pilates is an inspiring experience. To be sure it fits with your health objectives, first speak with your healthcare professional. Locate a peaceful, uncluttered area close to a sturdy wall. Give yourself a yoga mat and any extra gear you choose, such as resistance bands. For a strong foundation, concentrate on focused breathing, mild warm-ups, and foundational poses. Accept the wall's support while keeping a relaxed gait. Wall Pilates is a revitalizing way to increase strength, flexibility, and general well-being with little equipment needed and individual adaptations.

Setting up the Space

When engaging in Wall Pilates, it's important to set up the proper space, especially for seniors who might have certain requirements and considerations. Having a well-designed space during practice improves comfort, safety, and enjoyment in general. In this section, we'll go over the key components of creating the perfect environment for wall Pilates specific for seniors.

1. Open and Clear Space: First things first, make sure there is plenty of room for mobility and that the exercise area is clutter-free. Seniors ought to have unhindered movement in their arms and legs. Making the area clear reduces the possibility of mishaps and improves the Pilates routine's overall flow.

2. Robust Wall Support Point: Choose a wall that is sufficiently spacious to allow for the required exercises. The wall will function as a sturdy point of support for many kinds of motions. Make sure the wall is in good shape and has no protrusions or sharp edges that could be dangerous when performing activities.

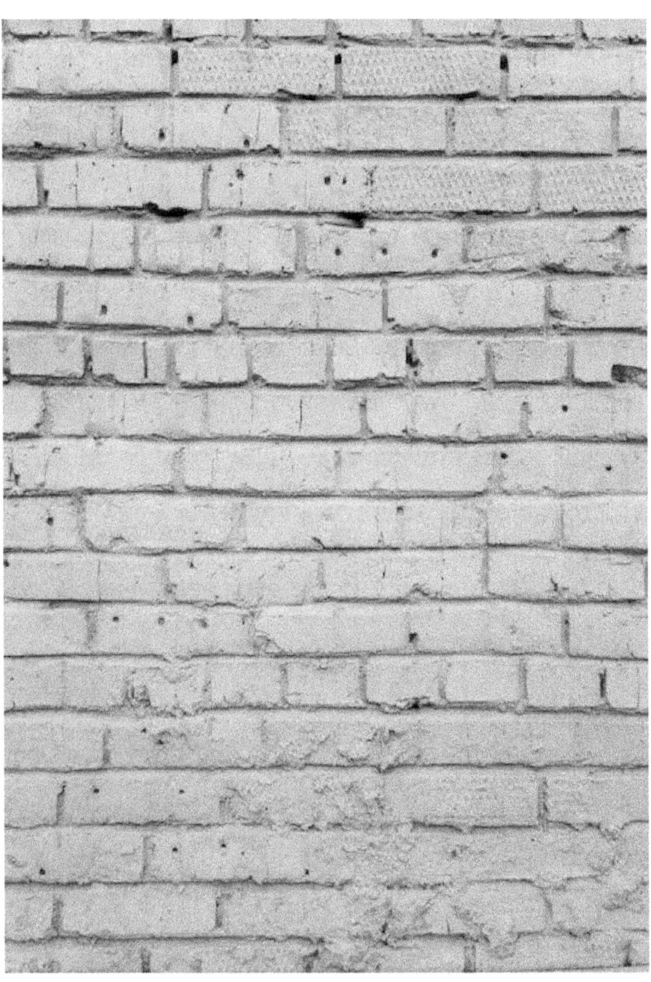

3. Comfortable Flooring: For seniors who need assistance with floor exercises or other activities that require sitting or lying down, choose a flooring surface that is both comfortable and non-slip. To give the spine and joints the necessary cushioning, use a yoga mat or cushioned workout mat.

4. Sufficient Lighting: Enough lighting is necessary for both vision and safety. Make sure there is adequate lighting in the workout area to prevent shadows and lower the chance of trips and falls. When accessible, natural light may produce a comfortable and welcoming ambiance.

5. Proper Ventilation: Keep your area well-ventilated to avoid overheating and guarantee a comfortable workout. Seniors doing Wall Pilates will find a more enjoyable setting when there is proper ventilation, which encourages the flow of fresh air.

6. Availability of Accessories and Props: Put any accessories or props that are required in a convenient location. This comprises straps, resistance bands, and any other tools needed for a particular activity.

Having these things close at hand makes working out easy and uninterrupted.

7. Personalized Modifications: Take into account each person's needs when arranging the area. Make sure that any extra assistance a participant needs, like a chair or handrails installed on the wall, is easily accessible. By making the environment flexible, individual adjustments can be made to meet the specific needs of every senior.

Necessary Equipment

A customized training program called wall Pilates is ideal for seniors over 50 who want to enhance their strength, flexibility, and balance while utilizing a sturdy wall for support. The simplicity of this method, which calls for little equipment, is what makes it so beautiful. The following is a thorough rundown of all the gear required to guarantee seniors have a fun, safe, and productive Wall Pilates experience:

1. Sturdy Wall: As the name implies, the basis of Wall Pilates is a sturdy and solid wall. Make sure the wall you have picked is clear of obstructions, kept up to date, and has enough room for all of your movements. Throughout the workouts, the wall provides stable support as a trustworthy anchor point.

2. An exercise mat or yoga mat: A surface that is both comfortable and non-slip is crucial for floor workouts and routines that require sitting or lying down. A yoga mat or exercise mat provides cushions to the joints and spine, improving comfort levels during the activity.

3. Resistance Bands: Resistance bands are a versatile and adjustable tool that provide a mild but effective level of resistance to a variety of workouts. They can be used by seniors to focus on particular muscle groups, increasing flexibility and strength without putting undue strain on their joints.

4. Pilates Straps: Pilate's straps are essential for supporting and guiding movements; they are frequently fastened to the wall. They lower the risk of strain while increasing accessibility to workouts by helping seniors maintain good form and alignment. The methodical and intentional quality of Pilate's movements is enhanced by the use of straps.

5. Soft Pilate's ball: Exercises become more varied when a soft Pilates ball is included, as it offers mild resistance. This apparatus is very useful for strengthening the core, enhancing stability generally, and improving balance. Seniors can hold and press the ball with comfort thanks to its smooth feel.

6. Comfy Clothes and Sneakers: Seniors should dress in loose-fitting, airy clothing that doesn't restrict their range of motion. Although most Wall Pilates exercises don't require shoes, those who would rather wear them during the class can choose supportive, non-slip versions.

7. Water Bottle: It's important to stay hydrated when doing any kind of workout. Seniors can maintain adequate hydration levels during their Wall Pilates practice by keeping a water bottle within reach, which promotes overall wellbeing.

8. Chair or Handrails (Optional): Depending on their particular requirements, seniors could gain from extra assistance. For individuals who need extra assistance or want the extra security, certain activities can be made more accessible with the help of a robust chair or wall-mounted handrails.

CHAPTER THREE
Warm-up Exercises

Any fitness program must begin with a warm-up, and wall Pilates for seniors over 50 is no different. These mild warm-up activities aim to enhance blood circulation, enhance range of motion, and prime the body for the forthcoming Wall Pilates practice. During these warm-ups, pay attention to your body and always prioritize appropriate form.

Neck Stretches

- Place your back on the wall while standing.

- Slowly tilt your head to the right, raising your ear toward your shoulder.

- Feel a slight stretch down the left side of your neck while you hold for 15 to 20 seconds.

- Repeat on the opposite side.

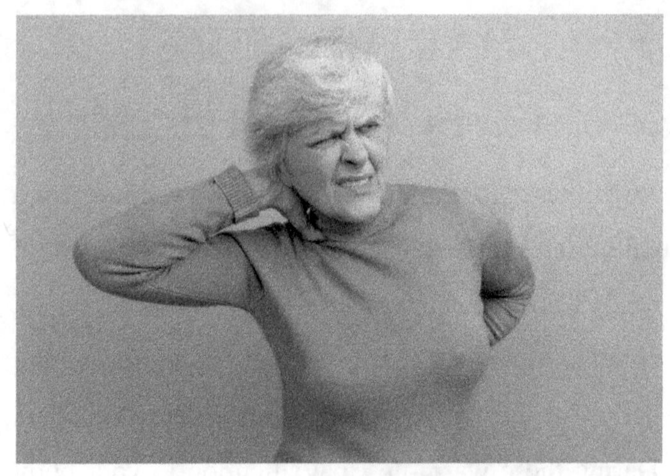

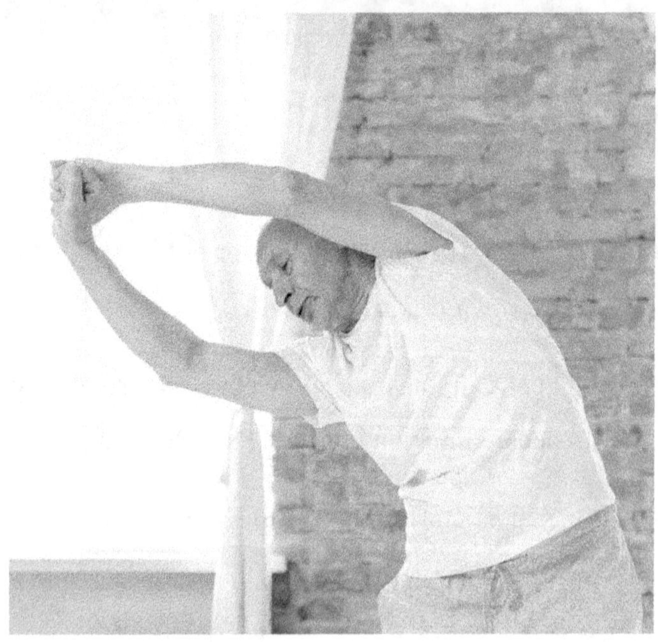

Shoulder Roll

- Stand tall with your feet shoulder-width apart.

- For ten repetitions, roll your shoulders forward in a circle.

- Turn around and roll your shoulders backward for an additional ten repetitions.

Arm Swing

- Stand and Place your feet hip-width apart.

- In a controlled manner, gently swing your arms forward and backward.

- As your muscles warm up, gradually extend your range of motion.

- 20 swings in each direction is the goal.

Spine Flexion

- Stand placing your hands at shoulder-height on the wall while facing the wall.

- Bending at the waist, slowly move your hands down the wall.

- Feel a light stretch along your spine as you hold the pose for 15 to 20 seconds.

- Move your hands back up the wall to get back to your starting position.

Hip Circles

- Stand placing your hands on your hips.

- Rotate your hips in a circular motion, making 10 circles in one direction.

- Make ten more circles in the opposite direction.

Lifts Your Knees

- Stand facing the wall and support yourself with your hands.

- Raise your right knee to your chest, hold it there for a little while, and then lower it.

- Repeat on your left knee.

- Try to lift 10 times on each leg.

Calf Raises

- Stand and place your hands on the wall for balance.

- Lift your heels off the ground and ascend onto your toes.

- Reposition your heels lower.

- Do 15 to 20 repetitions.

Ankle Circle

- Extend one leg while sitting on a chair or stand.

- Perform 10 repetitions of a circular ankle rotation in each direction.

- Do the same to the other leg.

Toe Taps

- Stand and Place your feet hip-width apart.

- Step forward and backward with your right toes.

- Repeat with your left foot.

- Tap each foot 20 more times.

Full Body Twist

- Stand and place your feet hip-width apart, arrange your arms in front of you.

- Swing your left hand across your body as you twist your torso to the right.

- Hold for a brief second before twisting to the left and extending your right hand.

- Twist 10 times on each side.

Taking Deep Breaths

After your warm-up, take a comfortable seat or stand. Breathe deeply through your nose, opening up your abdomen and chest. Breathe out slowly through your lips. To unwind physically and mentally before the Wall Pilates session, repeat these deep breathing exercises for two to three minutes.

CHAPTER FOUR
Foundation Wall Pilates Moves

Wall Roll Down

- Place your feet hip-width apart and stand with your back against the wall. Breathe in while tensing your abdomen.

- Release your breath and gently roll your spine, vertebral at a time, down the wall.

- When your spine is parallel to the floor, stop.

- Breathe in and raise yourself back to the starting position.

Wall Squats

- Position your feet shoulder-width apart and lean your back against the wall.

- Slide down the wall, bending your knees to a 90-degree angle.

- Make sure your ankles and knees are aligned.

- Hold for 10-15 seconds, then push through your heels to get back to the beginning position.

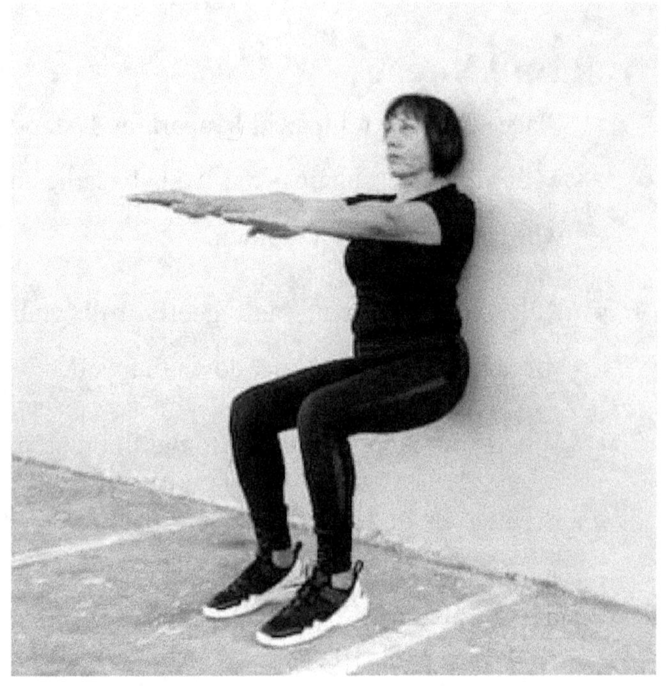

Leg Lifts

- Stand and face the wall, support yourself with your hands as you place it on it.

- Using your glutes, raise your right leg straight back.

- Hold for a moment before lowering.

- Proceed with the left leg.

- Try to lift ten times on each leg.

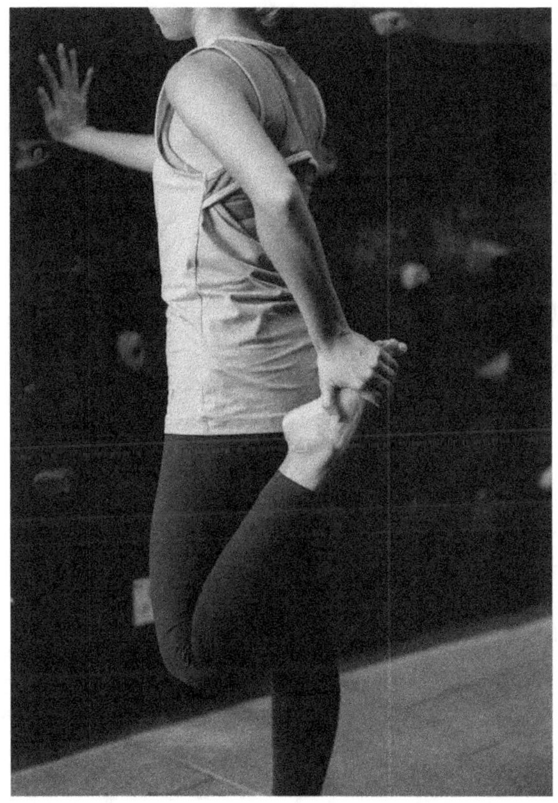

Wall Plank

- Face the wall and Place your hands shoulder
  height against the wall.

- Take a step back and straighten your body into a plank position.

- Maintain a straight posture while using your core.

- Hold for 20-30 seconds, extending the duration progressively as your strength increases.

Wall Bridge

- Lie on your back with your feet up against the wall, knees bent.

- Apply pressure to your heels, to raise your hips off the ground

- Hold the position for 15 to 20 seconds while using your core, then release it.

Wall Side Leg Lifts

- Place your hips up against the wall while lying on your side.

- Raise your upper leg straight up toward the ceiling.

- Reposition it so that it doesn't contact the lower leg.

- Do ten reps on each side.

Wall Chest Opener

- Stand facing the wall and put your hands shoulder-height on it.

- Take a step back and open your chest, stretching the front of your shoulders.

- Hold while inhaling deeply for 15 to 20 seconds.

One-leg wall stretch

- Place your hips toward the wall while lying on your back.

- Raise one leg and hold it with both hands toward the ceiling.

- Change legs in a controlled manner.

- Keep switching up the leg for 10 reps on each.

Arm Circles on Walls

- Stand with your side against the wall. Arm outstretched.

- Circle your arm forward for 10 repetitions, then change the direction.

- Change sides and repeat with the other arm.

Wall Chest Press

- Extend your arms while standing facing the wall.

- Using your chest muscles, press your palms toward the wall.

- Hold for 10-15 seconds, then release.

Breathe correctly and use controlled movements to complete these exercises. Increase the number of repetitions you do from the beginning as your strength and flexibility improve. Pay attention to your body and adjust the workouts as necessary to meet your fitness objectives and comfort level.

CHAPTER FIVE

Simple Wall Pilates Exercise to Improve Balance and Stability

These simple workouts are safe and efficient because they concentrate on strengthening the core and improving overall stability.

Wall Marching

Guidelines:

- Stand by putting your arms out in front of the wall.

- Put your hands shoulder-height on the wall.

- Raise your right knee to your chest, then lower it.

- March in place, alternating legs.

- For balance, engage your core.

- Try to complete 20 marches per leg.

Leg lift on wall plank

Guidelines:

- Stand facing the wall and place your hands shoulder-height on it.

- Take a step back and create a plank posture.

- Extend your right leg behind you by lifting it off the ground.

- Hold for a brief moment, then lower the leg.

- Lower the leg after a brief moment of holding.

- Repeat the same with your left leg.

- Elevate each leg 8-10 times

Toe Taps

Guidelines:

- Stand sideways towards the wall with your right shoulder facing it.

- Face your right shoulder toward the wall while standing sideways to it.

- Tap your right toes lightly against the wall and then tap them back.

- Use the left foot to the same.

- Move steadily while paying attention to your balance.

- Apply 15 taps on each foot.

Side Leg Lift

Guidelines:

- Stand and face the wall with your right side.

- For support, place your right hand against the wall.

- Raise your left leg to the side, then lower.

- Keep your posture straight.

- Repeat on the opposite side.

- Try to lift 10 times on each side.

Heel Raises

Guidelines:

- Place your back against the wall while standing.

- Raise your heels off the ground, rising onto the balls of your feet.

- Hold for a moment, then release your heels.

- Pay attention to control movement.

- Do 15-20 repetitions.

Single Leg Balance

Guidelines:

- Stand and face the wall, arms-length away

- Raise your right foot from the floor.

- Maintain the position for 15 to 20 seconds.

- Release the foot and Switch to the left.

- On each leg, repeat for three rounds.

Wall Squats

Guidelines:

- Place your back against the wall while standing.

- Slide down the wall and bend your knees to a 45-degree position.

- Hold for 15-20 seconds.

- To go back to your starting point, push through your heels.

- Do 2 to 3 sets.

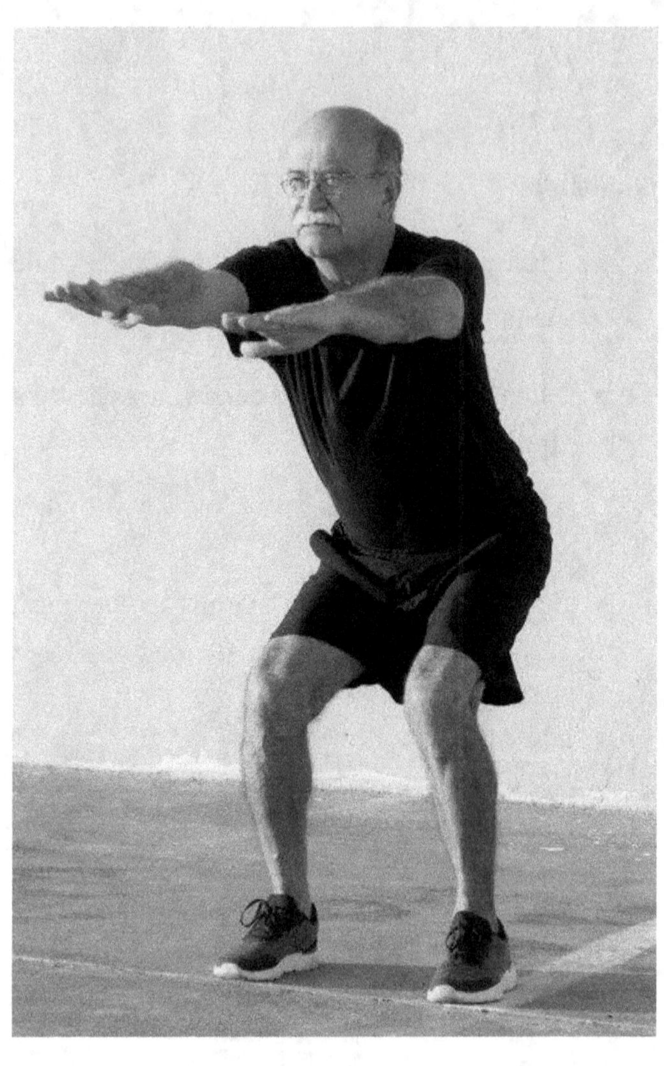

Knee Lifts with Rotation

Guidelines:

- Take a stand facing the wall and support yourself with your hands.

- Raise the right knee up towards your chest.

- Turn your torso in the direction of your raised knee.

- Lower the knee and repeat on the left side.

- Try to complete 10 turns on each side.

Wall Calf Stretch

Guidelines:

- Stand and face the wall and support yourself with your hands.

- Move back using your right foot, keeping the heel on the ground.

- Your right calf should feel stretched.

- Switch legs after 20 to 30 seconds of holding.

- Perform 2 rounds on each leg.

Hip Hinge

Guidelines:

- Stand facing the wall and Place your feet hip-width apart.

- Put your hands shoulder-height on the wall.

- Hinge at your hips, Push them back.

- Keep your back straight and chest raised.

- Return to a standing position again.

- Do this 15 to 20 repetitions.

CHAPTER SIX

Unique Wall Pilates for Flexibility and Range of Motion

Wall Hip Flexor Stretch

Guidelines:

- Stand facing the wall, arms-length away.

- Place your right foot against the wall behind you.

- Lean forward slightly while maintaining a straight back leg.

- Sensate the strain in your right hip's front.

- Switch legs after 20 to 30 seconds of holding.

Arm Circle Wall Chest Opener

Guidelines:

- Stand and face the wall, rest your right hand shoulder-height on it.

- Open your chest by rotating your torso away from the wall.

- Stretch your left arm out and rotate it in both directions in tiny circles.

- Repeat on the opposite side.

- Complete 10 rounds in each direction on each side.

Wall Cat-Cow Stretch

Guidelines:

- Stand by putting your arms out in front of the wall.

- Put your hands shoulder-height on the wall.

- Breathe in, lowering your abdomen and arching your back.

- Breathe out, tucking your chin in and rounding your back.

- Perform 8 to 10 repetitions of the flowing motion.

Wall Figure Four Stretch

Guidelines:

- Stand by putting your arms out in front of the wall.

- Raise your right foot to hip height and plant it on the wall.

- Sinking into a small squat by bending your left knee.

- Feel the strain in your glutes and right hip.

- Switch legs after 20 to 30 seconds of holding.

Wall Lateral Leg Swing

Guidelines:

- Take a sideways position against the wall and place your right hand on it for support.

- Laterally swing your left leg, crossing it in front of your body.

- Go back to the starting position.

- Perform 10 swings with each leg.

Mermaid Stretch on the Wall

Guidelines:

- Take a seat with your right side against the wall.

- Position your left hand on the ground and your right hand on the wall.

- Raise your hips off the ground, to create a side stretch.

- Switch sides after holding for 20 to 30 seconds.

Wall Spine Twist

Guidelines:

- Place your feet hip-width apart, Stand and face the wall.

- Place your hands shoulder-height on the wall.

- Rotate your torso to the right, reaching your right hand back.

- Switch sides after holding for 15 to 20 seconds.

Wall Hamstrings Stretch

Guidelines:

- Take a seat with your back against the wall and legs outstretched.

- Hinge at your hips and reach towards your toes.

- Feel the strain in your hamstrings as you hold for 20 to 30 seconds.

Wall Shoulders Opener

Guidelines:

- Stand by putting your arms out in front of the wall.

- Place your hands shoulder-height on the wall.

- Stretch your shoulders and chest by walking your hands down the wall.

- Hold for 20–30 seconds.

Wall Side Bend

Guidelines:

- Stand by putting your arms out in front of the wall.

- Bend to the left and extend your right arm along the wall.

- Feel the strain running down your right side.

- Switch sides after holding for 20 to 30 seconds.

Regularly perform these wall Pilates exercises to increase range of motion and flexibility. During each stretch, concentrate on making deliberate, fluid motions while taking deep breaths. Step up the intensity according to your comfort level, and as your flexibility improves, go faster.

CHAPTER SEVEN

Unique Wall Pilates Exercise to Cool Down and Relaxation

Wall Supported Forward Fold

Guidelines:

- Stand facing the wall, assume an arms-length away.

- Put your hands shoulder-height on the wall.

- Take a deep breath stretching your Spine.

- Release your breath and hinge at your hips, folding forward.

- Let your head relax, notice a gentle stretch in your hamstrings and lower back.

- Hold while taking deep breaths for 30 seconds.

- Carefully return to a standing position.

Deep Breathing Wall Chest Opener

Guidelines:

- Stand sideways to the wall, with your right hand at shoulder height on it.

- Open your chest by rotating your torso away from the wall.

- Take a deep breath, expanding your chest.

- Breathe out slowly while noticing how your shoulders and chest are stretched.

- Hold while taking steady, deep breaths for 20 seconds.

- Change sides, then perform the stretch again on your left side.

Seated Wall Spinal Twist

Guidelines:

- Place your right side up against the wall while seated on the floor.

- Bend your knees and Place your feet level on the ground.

- Touch the wall behind you with your right hand.

- Inhale, lengthen your spine, and twist to the right.

- Breathe out, feeling the strain in your spine and intensifying the twist.

- Hold while breathing steadily for 30 seconds.

- Change sides, then perform the stretch again on your left side.

Wall Pilates Butterfly Stretch

Guidelines:

- Sit close to the wall, position your back against it.

- Allow your knees to drop to the sides as you bring the soles of your feet together.

- Put your hands on your knees.

- Inhale as you expand your spine.

- Exhale and softly press your knees on the wall.

- Hold for 20 to 30 seconds, allowing your inner thighs to stretch.

- Take a deep breath and let the stretch release your tension.

Neck Tilt Stretch

Guidelines

- Place your feet hip-width apart and stand with your back to the wall.

- Tilt your head slightly to the right, putting your ear next to your shoulder.

- Feel a light stretch along the left side of your neck as you hold the pose for 15 seconds.

- Repeat with the left side.

Neck Rotation Stretch

Guidelines:

- Face the wall then turn your head to the right, bringing your chin to your shoulder.

- Hold while noticing the stretch in your neck for 15 seconds.

- Repeat with the left side.

Wall Supported Child's Pose

Guidelines:

- Kneel on the floor, face the wall with your big toes touching.

- Extend your arms forward and rest your hands against the wall while seated back on your heels.

- Place your forehead to rest on the wall feeling the strain along your spine.

- Hold while taking deep breaths for 30 seconds.

Seated Wall Twist

Guidelines:

- Sit against the wall and Place your legs out in front of you.

- Bend your right knee and Place your right foot on the outside of your left knee.

- Place your left elbow on the outside of your right knee and gently twist to the right.

- Hold for 15-20 seconds, feel the soft twist and the stretch in your spine.

- Repeat on the opposite side

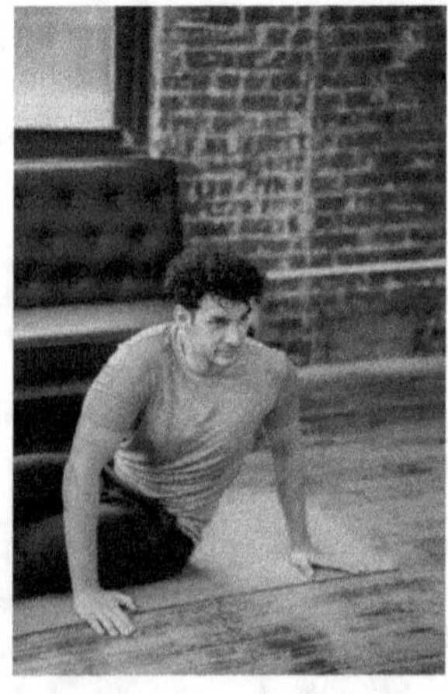

Addressing Common Challenges and Solutions for Seniors

For seniors over 50, starting a wall Pilates fitness adventure is a praiseworthy decision. Even though there are many advantages, it's important to recognize and deal with common issues that could come up during the practice. The goal of this book is to give seniors practical ways to deal with these obstacles so they can practice wall Pilates in safety and enjoyment.

Challenge 1: Insufficient Flexibility

Problem: Due to diminished flexibility, seniors may find it difficult to complete certain exercises to their full range of motion.

Solution: Incorporate light mobility exercises and dynamic stretches gradually into the warm-up regimen. To increase flexibility over time, concentrate on deliberate motions and promote regular practice.

Challenge 2: Joint Discomfort

Problem: Joint pain or discomfort may be experienced among seniors, particularly during weight-bearing activities.

Solution: Exercises should be modified to lessen impact and joint stress. Select low-impact versions and give joint health-supporting exercises first priority. Additionally, to be sure that workouts are safe for certain illnesses, speak with a healthcare provider.

Challenge 3: Problems with Balance

Problem: It can be challenging to maintain balance when performing wall Pilates exercises, particularly for seniors who may have stability issues.

Solution: Start with exercises that provide you more support, such as holding onto the wall or a strong chair. As your balance gets better, gradually go on to more difficult exercises. Include targeted balancing exercises in the routine to directly treat this issue.

Challenge 4: Muscle Weakness

Problem: Muscle weakness can be a problem for seniors, which can make it difficult for them to do some Pilates movements properly.

Solution: Include strength-training activities that focus on your main muscle groups. As strength increases, start with minimal resistance and progressively increase. Adapting workout intensity to each person's level of ability guarantees a safe and gradual method.

Challenge 5: Injury Fear

Problem: Seniors' reluctance to try new movements during Pilates exercises can be attributed to fear of injury.

Solution: Prioritize using the right form and technique for every exercise. Follow precise directions and promote a calm, steady pace. Reducing the fear of injury and fostering confidence are achieved through demonstrating changes and providing a supportive environment.

Challenge 6: Lack of Motivation

Problem: Difficulties may set in for seniors to stay motivated to practice Pilates regularly.

Solution: To keep the routine interesting, add variety. Establish reasonable objectives and acknowledge success. Finding a workout partner or enrolling in group programs can also offer a social component, which improves accountability and motivation.

Challenge 7: Time Restriction

Problem: Due to numerous obligations, seniors might find it difficult to find time for a regular Pilates practice.

Solution: Create brief, efficient routines that fit into daily schedules with ease. Stress the value of consistency over length and offer options for brief but effective sessions.

Challenge 8: Difficulty in Breathing

Problem: A senior's ability to efficiently do exercises may be impacted by their inability to coordinate breath with movement.

Solution: Make breath awareness your top priority and use targeted breathing techniques in your warm-up. Seniors should encouraged to concentrate on breathing during the preparation stage of each exercise and out during the effort period.

Challenge 9: Space Restriction

Problem: Several people may not have much room for exercise, which makes it difficult to execute several Pilates exercises.

Solution: Adapt workouts to fit the available area. Pay attention to motions that can be executed in a small space. In order to meet different spatial constraints, offer choices that can be completed while seated or standing.

Challenge 10: Intimidation with New Movements

Problem: Seniors who are afraid of the unfamiliarity of Pilates exercises may find it intimidating to try new motions.

Solution: Begin with basic exercises and work your way up to more difficult ones. To increase confidence, highlight the learning process and acknowledge minor accomplishments. Intimidation can be reduced by fostering a positive and encouraging environment.

Seniors can confidently reap the many advantages of wall Pilates by addressing these typical problems and receiving customized solutions, which makes wall Pilates a rewarding and affordable training choice for people over 50. Prioritize your personal needs and safety above all else when you workout.

CONCLUSION

In summary, Wall Pilates is a life-changing experience for adults over 50 that goes beyond a simple workout regimen. It is a dedication to improved health, vigor, and strength. After delving into the different aspects of Wall Pilates, including its distinctive exercises, difficulties, and the soothing techniques of guided relaxation and cool-downs, it is clear that this type of exercise is a comprehensive strategy designed to meet the particular requirements of the elderly population.

The versatility of Wall Pilates is just as important as its physical advantages. It embraces the wide range of skills and difficulties that seniors could experience. Seniors can progressively increase their strength, flexibility, and feeling of stability and balance with safe, effective workouts.

We've addressed the common challenges that may arise, providing thoughtful solutions to ensure a safe and enjoyable fitness journey.

Whether it's addressing joint discomfort, enhancing flexibility, or overcoming any initial hesitation, Wall Pilates offers a customizable and accommodating path to health.

The cool-down and relaxation techniques that are offered address the significance of recuperation and mental health, acknowledging that true fitness is a combination of physical and mental health. The breathing exercises and guided relaxation techniques promote the development of a calm and focused state of mind in addition to the release of physical stress.

Seniors who practice Wall Pilates take up a lifestyle that emphasizes self-care, awareness, and the pursuit of long-term health, rather than merely a set of exercises. This method encourages a healthy connections between the body and mind by going beyond conventional ideas of exercise

For seniors over 50, Wall Pilates is essentially an invitation to rediscover the joy of movement, to honor the body's resiliency, and to bask in the feeling of achievement that comes with each customized workout. It's a dedication to growing older with grace, resilience, and a spirit that knows no bounds.

Thus, let the wall serve as your constant traveling companion—a scaffolding that promotes advancement and a blank canvas for you to draw the picture of your own wellbeing. The wall is there to support, encourage, and celebrate each step you take toward becoming a healthier, more energetic version of yourself, regardless of how experienced you are with Pilates.

You choose the path to take, and there are countless opportunities for reviving and vigor with Wall Pilates. We wish you strength, balance, and the achievement of your fitness goals in the future.

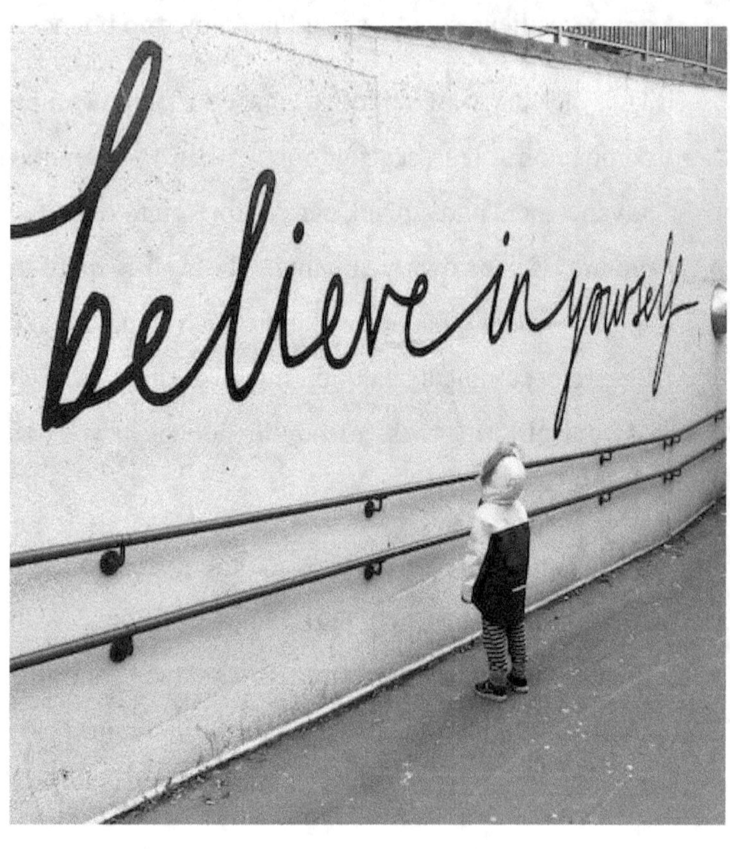
believe in yourself

PART II: CHAIR EXERCISE FOR SENIORS OVER 50

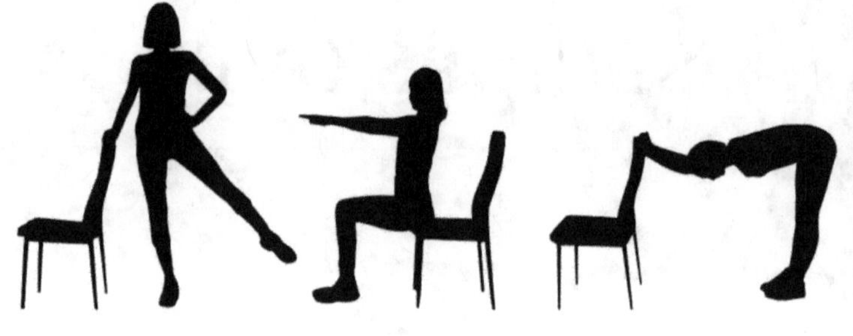

INTRODUCTION

The value of embracing vitality transcends age, as each thread in the tapestry of life tells the tale of our journey. The idea of exercise becomes more than just a choice as we approach our golden years; it becomes a necessary partner in our pursuit of resilience and good health. Chair exercise is a beacon for people over 50, beckoning them to a sanctuary of movement that transcends age, by unveiling a world where energy meets experience.

Imagine a situation in which the cadence of the muscles involved in a dance of well-being and the rhythm of life are in harmony. This is the fundamental element of **chair exercise for seniors over 50**—a motion symphony that surpasses the constraints of conventional exercise regimens. Moving beyond the practicality of mobility, it becomes an empowerment story, supporting the idea that growing older is a step toward a fuller, more engaged life rather than a step back.

Meet Arthur whose life unfolded, a melody of golden years that, at first, played a tune of weariness and body weakness. The mirror reflected a silhouette overshadowed by the ghost of vitality past, and fatigue seemed a constant companion. However, within this quiet surrender, Arthur discovered a tenacity that lay dormant.

Enter the protagonist—a chair. Not just a resting place, but a vessel for transformation. Arthur's journey into rejuvenation began with the rhythmic cadence of seated movements. The chair, once a passive piece of furniture, now became the conduit to revival. Lift by lift, stretch by stretch, it morphed into a throne of triumph.

As weeks turned into months, Arthur's narrative transformed into a vibrant tapestry of resilience. The chair, once underestimated, emerged as a catalyst for change, and exercise, the elixir that breathed life into tired muscles.

The weariness that had cast its shadow gave way to a newfound energy humming through his days. This is not merely Arthur's story; it's a universal journey, an invitation to rediscover the vitality lingering within. As we explore the pages of **"Chair Exercise for Seniors Over 50**," let Arthur's tale be a testament to the transformative power of a seemingly simple act. The chair, with its silent strength, invites everyone to engage in a dance of rejuvenation—one lift, one stretch, one triumph over time at a time.

In these pages, discover the chair not as a symbol of repose but as a companion in the quest for flourishing beyond 50, proving that the chapters of life can be rewritten with every intentional movement, and the chair becomes not just a seat but a throne of renewed vigor.

We are going to go beyond the traditional notion of physical activity as we explore the world of chair exercise. It's an ode to tenacity, a choreography of sitting motions that reveals inner potential and demonstrates that the joy of movement should not be limited to the strenuous activities of the youthful and joyful. This is a tribute to the understanding that recognizes the symbiotic relationship between the body and the chair—a relationship that liberates rather than restricts, encouraging strength and agility in each lifted and stretched pose while seated.

Join the movement as a meaningful demonstration of the resolve to age gracefully and to seize every chance for vitality, not simply in the literal sense. Chair exercise is not a trade-off; rather, it's a revelation that opens a portal to a universe in which youth is but a number and the soul, eternally youthful, moves to the beat of good health. The chair takes on a new role in life after 50, serving as a throne of exercise and metamorphosis as well as a royal edict that declares, "Thou shalt flourish!"

Benefits of Chair Exercise for Seniors

In the dynamic symphony of aging gracefully, the chair—often overlooked—becomes a potent ally for seniors over 50 seeking to maintain their health and energy. Chair exercises are easy to do and very accessible. They can be a life-changing experience with many advantages that go beyond typical workout regimens. Let's examine the many benefits that make chair workouts an essential component of fostering health and stamina in later life.

1. Strengthens Muscular Tissue: For elders, chair exercises offer a gentle yet efficient way to increase muscle strength. Individuals can work different muscle groups, improving tone and resilience, with deliberate motions and exercises. This promotes independence by helping with daily tasks and improving mobility at the same time.

2. Enhances Heart Health: Despite the common notion that high impact exercise is necessary for optimal cardiovascular exercise, chair workouts provide a heart-healthy substitute. Engaging in Seated aerobic exercise raises heart rate and improves cardiovascular endurance and circulation. This helps to improve stamina and heart health in general.

3. Increases Range of Motion and Flexibility: Chair exercises help with the frequent issues of stiffness that come with age by facilitating a gradual increase in range of motion and flexibility. Joint mobility is increased through stretching and deliberate movement, which also reduces pain and improves total motion fluidity.

4. Promotes Stability and Balance: Seniors are more likely to stumble because they frequently struggle with stability and balance. Chair workouts that include seated balance routines strengthen and stabilize the core muscles. This builds confidence in everyday movements and makes a substantial contribution to fall prevention.

5. Controls Metabolism and Weight: As one ages, maintaining a healthy weight becomes more and more important. Chair workouts help burn calories and maintain lean muscle mass when done on a regular basis. This helps to maintain a healthier metabolism in addition to helping with weight management.

6. Reduces Joint Discomfort: Arthritis and other joint disorders commonly cause discomfort in seniors. Chair exercises are a low-impact way to reduce joint stress and increase joint strength and flexibility. This makes it the perfect alternative for those looking for low-impact exercise options.

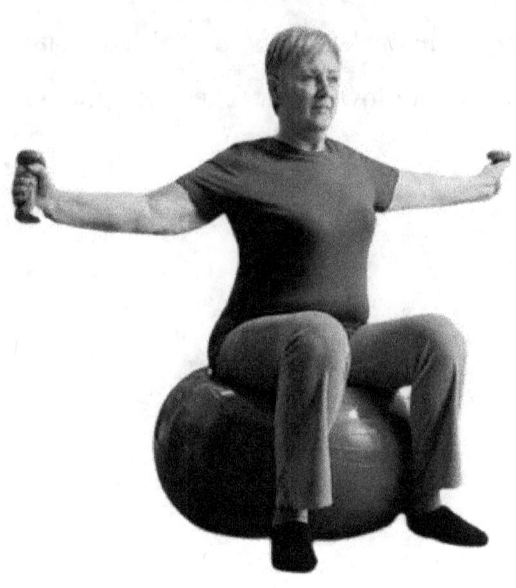

CHAPTER ONE
Setting Up Your Chair Exercise Space

Chair exercise is a flexible and inclusive type of physical activity that may be done by anyone, regardless of fitness or mobility level. It is meant to be done while seated. The idea is to perform a series of exercises while seated on a chair in order to activate various muscle groups and increase flexibility. A wide range of individuals can benefit from these exercises, such as elderly people, people with restricted mobility, and people healing from injuries.

The versatility of chair exercise is what makes it so beautiful. It covers a range of fitness levels with motions that include strength-building and sitting aerobics as well as soothing stretches. This method takes into account the psychological advantages of maintaining an active lifestyle, which promotes a sense of independence and accomplishment, in addition to the participants' physical well-being.

Chair exercises can be included into a regular exercise program or used as an adjunctive activity to improve cardiovascular health, muscular strength, and flexibility. The chair, a fundamental component of inclusive fitness, evolves from a simple seat to an empowerment tool that enables people of all ages and physical abilities to start their path toward well-being. Chair exercise essentially represents the idea that health may be developed in the most accessible and accommodating environments and that movement has no boundaries.

Creating a Safe and Comfortable Environment

As we embark on the journey of chair exercise for seniors, it is crucial to create a space that not only encourages safety but also comfort and self-assurance.

Optimizing the environment to meet the specific requirements of this group increases workout effectiveness and guarantees a good experience. Now let's explore the detailed procedures for setting up the perfect environment for chair workouts.

1. Select the Appropriate Chair: Choosing the right chair is essential to creating a secure workout space. Choose a supportive chair that has a backrest for extra support and a flat, non-slip surface. It should be possible to sit with your feet comfortably resting on the floor and maintain good posture.

2. Make Space Available: Make sure there is enough space surrounding the chair in a designated workout area. In order to create a space that is safe and clear for movement, remove any potential barriers or tripping risks. Make sure there are no loose objects on the floor and that any carpets or rugs are fastened to avoid slipping.

3. Sufficient Lighting: Having a well-lit environment is essential for safety, particularly when exercising. To lower the chance of tripping or falling, make sure the exercise environment is well-lit. While natural light is best, powerful artificial lighting can be used in its place if it's unavailable.

4. Customized Adjustments: Acknowledge each participant's unique demands and adjust as needed. For further comfort and support if needed, think about adding cushions or pillows. Customize the experience to take into account any health issues or physical restrictions.

5. Warm Up and Cool Down Areas: Set aside particular spaces for your warm-up and cool-down activities. This promotes flexibility and avoids sudden movements that could cause discomfort or injury by enabling participants to flow fluidly between the various workout phases.

6. Sufficient Air Circulation: To guarantee that participants stay comfortable during the whole workout program, keep the area well-ventilated. Enough airflow keeps things from getting too hot and creates a more comfortable atmosphere overall.

7. Equipment and Props That Are Accessible: Make sure props and equipment are easily accessible while using them. Chair workouts can be made more interesting by using resistance bands, small weights, or exercise balls. But these have to be accessible, and users have to know how to utilize them.

8. Educational Images: Present lucid and succinct educational graphics. Exercise posters or charts with instructions on how to perform each exercise properly can be quite helpful, especially for people who are not familiar with chair exercises. This improves comprehension and lowers the possibility of mis-executing motions.

9. Supportive Community: Encourage a feeling of camaraderie and assistance among involved parties. To promote conversation and unity, arrange chairs in a circle. This improves chair exercises' social component and fosters an upbeat, inspiring environment.

10. Continual Safety Inspections: Make routine safety inspections of the equipment and workout space. Make sure the flooring is in good shape, the lighting fixtures work, and the chairs stay firm. Regular evaluations help maintain a consistently safe atmosphere.

Necessary Equipment and Props

Chair exercises for seniors offer a gentle yet effective way to promote health and well-being, and incorporating the correct equipment and props can enhance the experience and benefits of these workouts. Here's a brief overview to the necessary equipment for a chair exercise routine specific to seniors.

1. Robust Chair: Choosing a robust chair with a flat, non-slip surface and a supportive backrest is the cornerstone of chair workouts. The height of the chair should enable users to sit with their feet comfortably resting on the floor and retain good posture.

2. Resistance Straps: Chair workouts benefit greatly from the addition of resistance bands, which offer mild resistance to help build muscles. They are particularly helpful for increasing the flexibility and strength of the upper body. To accommodate different levels of fitness, select bands with variable resistance levels.

Light Weights: Adding dumbbells or modest weights to chair workouts increases muscle strength. Choose weights that are easy to handle and offer a challenge without being too taxing. As your strength grows, progressively increase the weight you start with.

4. Exercise Ball: You can use an exercise ball to work your core muscles and perform stability exercises. Ball exercises that are done while seated can improve flexibility and balance. Make sure the ball is the right size so that participants can stay stable while seated.

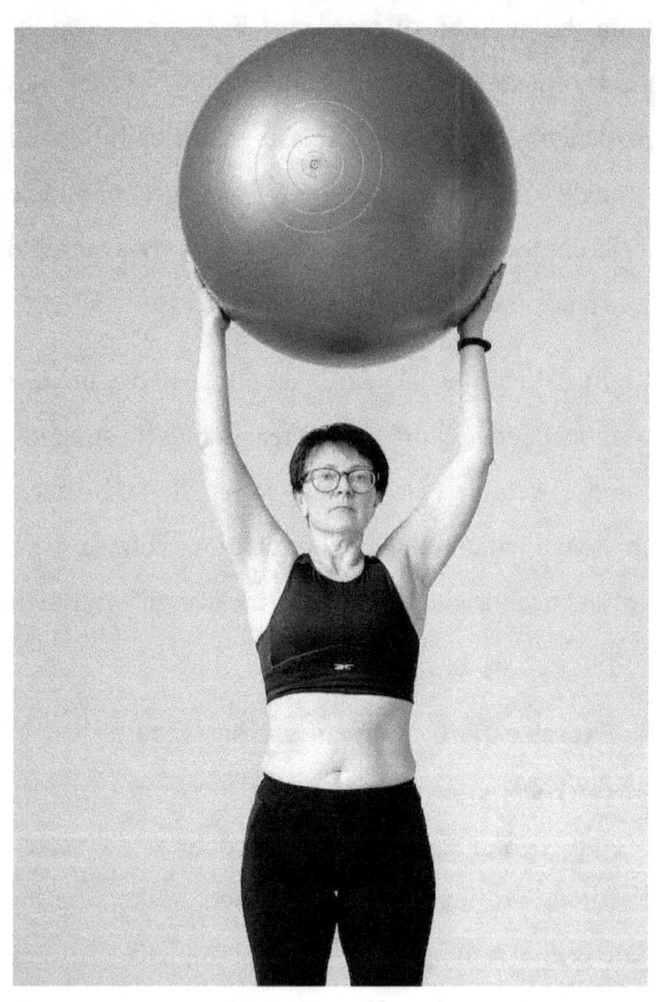

5. Pillows or cushions: Provide cushions or pillows to offer extra support to improve comfort. It is possible to reduce pressure points and enhance comfort by placing them strategically, which is especially beneficial for people who have joint sensitivity.

6. Yoga Straps: Yoga straps are useful equipment for stretches and flexibility training. They let people reach their full range of motion with moderate assistance without sacrificing safety. Straps are very helpful for seniors who are trying to become more flexible.

7. Stability Discs: By adding an element of instability, stability discs placed on the chair seat might make it harder for users to maintain their balance by using their core muscles. This small addition keeps things low-impact and joint-friendly while adding intensity to the workout.

8. Graphic Aids for Instruction: Exercises can be facilitated by using simple, instructive graphics, such charts or posters. In order to ensure proper form and technique, visual aids are very important for people who may be new to chair exercises.

9. Clock or Timer: Include a clock or timer in the program to assist participants in keeping track of how long the exercises and rest periods last. Participants are encouraged to advance at their own rate and an organized workout atmosphere is created as a result.

Safety Tips and Guidelines for Safe Chair Exercise

For seniors, starting a chair exercise regimen can be a fulfilling experience that fosters health and energy. Following these safety advice and guidelines is essential to a fun and safe experience:

1. Speak with a Healthcare Professional: Speak with your healthcare provider before beginning any new fitness regimen, particularly if you have any underlying medical ailments or concerns. They can provide tailored guidance according to your particular requirements.

2. Pick a Stable Chair: Choose a sturdy chair with a supportive backrest and a flat, non-slip surface. For optimal posture during workouts, the chair's height should enable your feet to rest comfortably on the floor.

3. Warm-Up and Cool Down: Always start with a light warm-up to get the joints and muscles ready for action. Similarly, cool down at the end of your activity to gradually reduce heart rate and avoid stiffness.

4. Initiate Slowly and Advance Gradually: Start with simple workouts and low resistance, as your strength increases, progressively increase the intensity of your workouts. By taking a stepwise approach, you lower your chance of injury and give your body time to adjust to the new habit.

5. Maintain Proper Posture: Sit up straight with your shoulders relaxed and core tight. Maintaining good posture not only makes exercises more effective but also lessens the risk of neck and back injury.

6. Listen to Your Body: Observe how your body feels both during and after physical activity. In case you encounter any pain, lightheadedness, or peculiar unease, discontinue the exercise immediately and seek advice from your physician.

7. Stay Hydrated: Throughout your workout, have a water bottle close by and stay hydrated. Staying well hydrated is crucial for general health, particularly while engaging in strenuous exercise.

8. Refrain from Overexerting Yourself: Although it's good to push yourself, don't push yourself too far to the point of weariness. Building strength without running the danger of injury requires gradual improvement.

9. Use Appropriate Equipment: Make sure any props or weights you use are in good shape and suitable for your level of fitness. For chair exercises, resistance bands and small weights are popular options.

10. Create a Safe Exercise Space: Remove any possible trip hazards from the space surrounding your chair. To provide a safe environment for exercising, make sure there is adequate lighting and ventilation.

11. Incorporate Breathing Techniques: Throughout your exercises, concentrate on maintaining a steady, controlled breathing pattern. Breathing correctly increases oxygen flow, which encourages relaxation and endurance.

12. Be Aware of Current Conditions: Adjust your workouts to account for any particular health issues you may have. For example, people with arthritis may decide to engage in low-impact activities in order to preserve their joints.

13. Engage in Regular Health Check-Ups: Discuss your workout regimen with your doctor on a regular basis to make sure it is appropriate for your present state of health. Frequent evaluations assist in modifying the program to meet your changing needs.

Seniors who adhere to these safety precautions and instructions can reap the benefits of chair exercises while lowering their chance of harm. Recall that improving general well-being is the main objective, and a safe method guarantees a long-lasting and rewarding fitness adventure.

CHAPTER TWO
Warm-Up Routine

Seated Neck Tilts

- Take a comfortable seat with your back straight.

- Slowly tilt your head to the right, lowering your ear to your shoulder.

- Feel a light stretch along the left side of your neck as you hold for 10-15 seconds.

- Repeat with the left side. Execute two sets on each side.

Shoulder Rolls

- Sit up straight and place your feet flat on the floor.

- Roll your shoulders up, back, down, and forward in a circular motion.

- Repeat for 15 to 20 seconds, then change to the other direction.

- This exercise increases mobility and helps release shoulder muscles.

Seated Side Bends

- Sit up straight and keep your feet flat on the ground.

- Gently tilt to one side, feeling a stretch along your waist.

- Return to the center after holding for 10 seconds.

- Repeat on the opposite side. Execute 2 sets on each side.

Ankle Circles

- Raise one foot a little off the floor and turn your ankle in a clockwise direction.

- Make ten circles in a single direction, then switch counterclockwise.

- Continue with the other foot.

- Ankle circles warm up the muscles in the lower legs and increase ankle flexibility.

Seated Marching

- Take a seat with good and bring one knee up to your chest.

- Lower it down, then switch to the other knee to repeat.

- Keep marching for 30 seconds.

- This exercise increases circulation and engages the hip flexors.

Seated Torso Twist

- Place your hands on the opposing edges of your chair while sitting upright.

- Twist your torso gently to one side, then hold it there for 10 seconds.

- Return to the center and repeat on the opposite side.

- Perform two sets on each side to warm up the spine.

Extensor Stretch and Wrist Flexor

- Extend your arm, with the palm facing down.

- To stretch the wrist flexors, lightly press down on the fingers with the opposing hand.

- After holding for 10 seconds, raise your palm up, stretching your wrist extensors.

- Repeat on both arms to improve wrist mobility.

Seated Leg Swings

- Take a seat on the chair's edge and extend one leg forward.

- Gently swing your leg back and forth, increasing the range of motion.

- Execute for 15 seconds, then move to the other legs.

- Leg swings improve leg mobility and warm up the hip flexors.

Chest Opener

- Take a seat tall and put your hands behind your back.

- Raise your arms slightly, forcing your shoulder blades together and opening your chest.

- Hold for 10 seconds then release.

- This exercise improves chest mobility and combats slouching.

Diaphragmatic Breathing While Seated

- Sit comfortably and Put your hands on your belly.

- Take a deep breath through your nose, expanding your diaphragm.

- Slowly release air with pursed lips while engaging your core.

- Repeat for a minute to encourage mental clarity and relaxation.

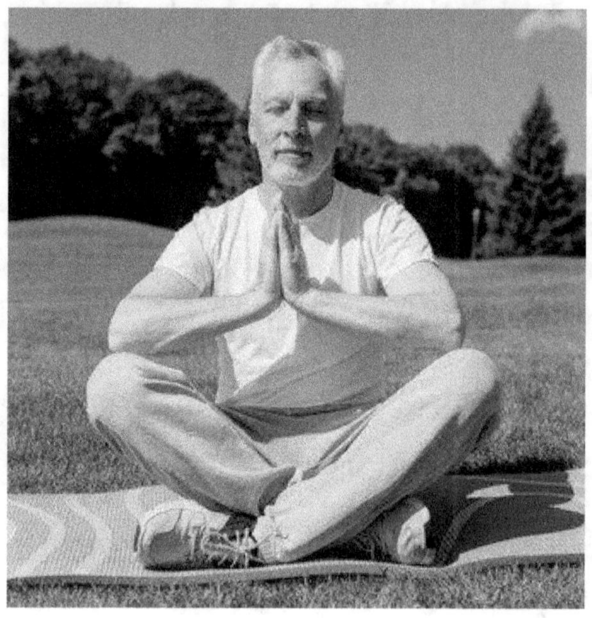

CHAPTER THREE
Simple Upper Body Chair Exercises

Seated Arm Raises

- Sit with your back straight and place your feet flat on the ground.

- Breathe in and extend both arms straight in front of you, pointing upward the ceiling.

- Breathe out and bring your arms back down.

- To strengthen shoulders and increase range of motion, repeat for 15 repetitions.

Chair Dips

- Take a seat on the chair's edge and hold onto the front edge with your hands.

- Slide forward until your hips are barely off the chair.

- Bend your elbows and lower your body a few inches.

- Push back to return to the starting position.

- Perform for 12 reps to target the triceps and upper arms.

Sitting Shoulder Press

- Hold a light weight in each hand (or use water bottles).

- Lift the weights to shoulder height while maintaining a straight back seat.

- Arms extended, press the weights overhead.

- Reposition the weights back to shoulder height.

- To strengthen arms and shoulders, repeat for 12 reps.

Seated Rowing

- Use both hands to hold a resistance band in front of you.

- Sit erect and pull the strap toward your chest, squeezing your shoulder blades.

- Gently let go of the tension by spreading your arms.

- To target the muscles in the upper back, repeat for 15 reps.

Triceps Extensions

- Raise both hand overhead while holding one weight.

- Bend your elbows by lowering the weight behind your head.

- Arms straighten, lift the weight back up.

- Repeat for 12 reps to strengthen and tone triceps.

Seated Bicep Curls

- With your arms at your sides, hold a weight in each hand.

- Keep your elbows close to your body and Curl the weights in the direction of your shoulders.

- Gently lower the weights back down.

- To tone and engage the bicep muscles, repeat for 15 reps.

Seated Chest Press

- Bend your elbows 90 degrees, holding a weight in each hand.

- Press the weight forward, stretching your arms.

- Return the weights back to the starting position.

- Repeat 12 times to target the chest muscles.

CHAPTER FOUR
Chair Exercise to Strengthen Lower Body

Seated Leg Lifts

- Sit tall with feet level on the floor.

- Raise one leg straight forward and keep it there for 2 seconds.

- Lower it back down.

- Alternately perform 15 repetitions on each leg.

Heels Lift

- Place your feet hip-width apart and sit.

- Raise both heels off the ground.

- Hold for 3 seconds, then bring it down.

- Perform 20 reps to activate the calf muscles.

Seated March with Resistance Band

- Fasten a resistance band around your thighs.

- Sit upright and Lift one knee at a time.

- Step still for 30 seconds, feeling resistance.

- This strengthens the thighs and hips.

Seated Leg Press

- Position a little ball between your knees.

- Squeeze the ball while pressing your legs outward.

- Hold for 3 seconds, then release.

- Perform 15 reps to target the inner thighs.

Seated Knee Extensions

- Sit upright and extend one leg straight.

- Hold for 2 seconds then lower.

- Perform 12 reps on each leg to target the quadriceps.

Inner Squeeze of Thigh

- Put a cushioned ball in between your knees.

- Squeeze the ball using your inner thighs muscles.

- Hold for 5 seconds, then release.

- Repeat for 15 times to tone inner thighs.

Seated Hip Abduction

- Sit straight back and raise one knee to the side.

- Lower after 3 seconds of holding.

- Complete 12 repetitions on each side.

- This exercise works the hips' outer muscles.

Seated Hip Flexor Stretch

- Take a seat close to the chair's edge.

- Straighten one leg in front of you.

- Slightly bend forward, feeling your hips stretch.

- Switch legs after holding for 15 seconds.

Leg Circles with a Seat

- Stretch out one leg and use your foot to create little circles.

- Rotate in clockwise direction for 10 seconds, then counterclockwise.

- Change legs and repeat.

- This workout improves ankle range of motion.

Seated Hamstring Stretch

- Sit upright and extend one leg straight.

- Hinge at your hips, reaching for your toes.

- Hold for 15 seconds, or until your hamstrings start to stretch.

- Repeat with the opposite leg.

CHAPTER FIVE
Core-Strengthening Chair Exercises

Seated Marching with Torso Twist

- Place your feet flat on the ground and sit Upright.

- Raise one knee to your chest and twist your torso so the elbow on the other side comes close to the knee.

- Go back to the starting position and change sides.

- Repeat 15 reps on each side, working both the hip and core muscles.

Seated Leg Extensions with Abdominal Contraction

- Sit upright, constrict your abdominal muscles.

- Extend one leg straight in front of you.

- Switch legs after a few seconds of holding while using your core.

- Complete 12 reps on each leg, concentrating on controlled motions.

Seated Side Crunches

- Sit on the chair's edge and place your feet flat.

- Put one hand behind your head and raise the elbow so that it points toward the other knee.

- Go back to the beginning and change sides.

- Perform 15 reps on each side, focusing on your oblique.

Seated Russian Twists

- Sit up straight and use both hands to hold a medicine ball or light weight.

- Twist your torso to the right, then to the left, and pass the weight from one side to another.

- Twist 20 times, using your entire core.

Chair-Sided Cycling Crunches

- Sit back on the chair, lean back gently, and Raise your feet off the floor.

- Rotate your torso to touch your left elbow to your knee, and bring your right knee up to your chest.

- Change sides, making a motion similar to cycling.

- Repeat 15 reps on each side to target the entire core.

Seated Side Plank

- Sit on the chair's edge and put your right hand on the seat.

- Stretch your legs to the side, keeping a stack position.

- Raise your hips so that they create a side plank toward the ceiling.

- Hold for 20 seconds, then change sides.

Chair Plank with Knee Tucks

- Spread your legs back into a plank position while placing your hands on the chair's seat.

- Using your core, bring one leg up to your chest.

- Perform 15 knee tucks on each side, switching legs.

Seated V-Ups

- Sit upright, extending your legs and arms reaching towards the ceiling.

- Raise your torso and legs in a V-shape towards each other.

- Take a moment to hold, then release the pressure.

- Perform 12 reps, focusing on your entire core.

Seated Cow-Cow Stretch

- Sit upright putting your hands on your knees.

- Raise your head and arch your back while lowering your chest (Cow).

- Then, turn your back, bringing your chin to your chest (Cat).

- Repeat 10 times to increase spine flexibility.

Seated Torso Circles

- Sit upright and Put your hands on your hips.

- Turn your torso slowly to the right for 10 seconds, then back to the left.

- This dynamic exercise improves stability and flexibility in the core.

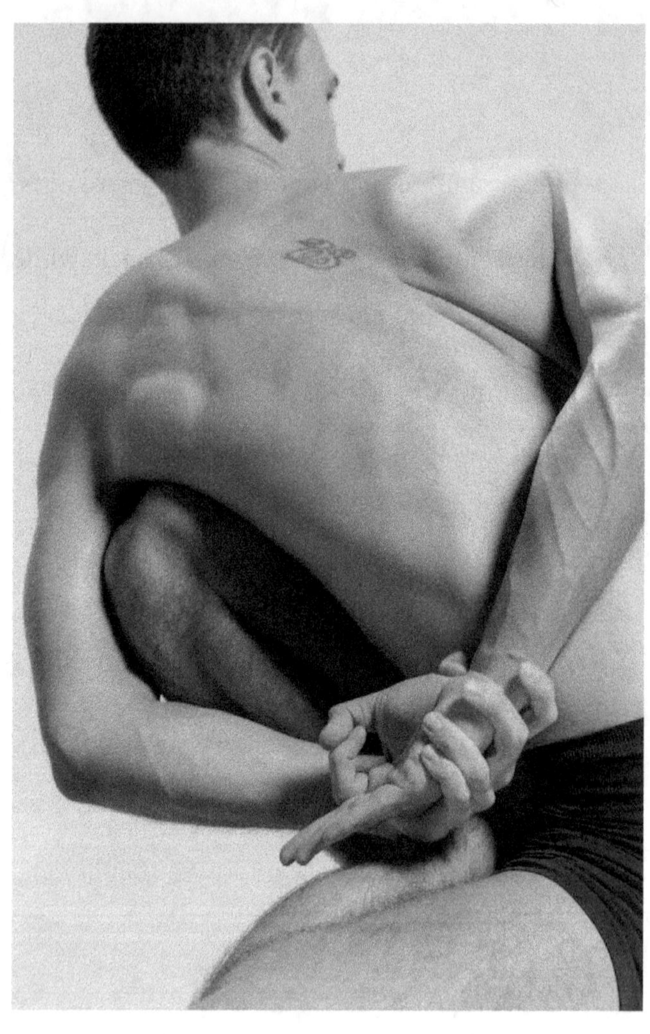

CHAPTER SIX
Cool-down and Relaxation Workouts

Seated Forward Fold

- Sit upright on the chair and Place your feet flat on the ground.

- Breathe in and lengthen your spine.

- Breathe out a hinge at your hips, extend towards your toes.

- Hold for 20 seconds, feeling slight stretch in your hamstrings and lower back.

Seated Side Stretch

- Take a comfortable seat and lift one arm overhead.

- Take a deep breath and extend your spine.

- Let out a breath and tilt slightly to the other side.

- Hold for 15 seconds, feeling the stretch along your side.

- Repeat on the opposite side.

Shoulder and Neck Rolls While Seated

- Sit upright and rotate your shoulders in circular motion.

- Breathe in as you raise them up and breathe out as you lower them back.

- Repeat for 30 seconds to ease shoulder and neck stiffness.

Deep Breathing Workout

- Sit comfortably, close your eyes, and lay one hand on your chest and the other on your abdomen.

- Take a deep breath through your nose, expanding your diaphragm

- Breathe out gently through pursed lips as you feel your abdomen drop.

- Continue for 2 minutes, encouraging rest and reducing tension in the body.

Seated Spinal Twist

- Sit with your feet flat on the floor and your back straight.

- Inhale and lengthen your spine.

- Exhale and twist slowly to one side, supporting yourself on the chair's back.

  Hold for 15 seconds, then move to the opposite side.

Meditation while seated

- Sit comfortably and put your hands on your knees.

- Close your eyes and pay attention to your breathing.

- Breathe in positivity, breathe out tension.

- Spend five minutes in meditation to promote mental calmness.

The goals of these relaxation and cool-down chair exercises for seniors over 50 are to increase flexibility, ease stress, and create a calming atmosphere. After your chair workout, try these movements to help your body and mind relax and reap the benefits of a mild cool down. Always proceed cautiously and carefully, and if you have any health problems, seek medical advice.

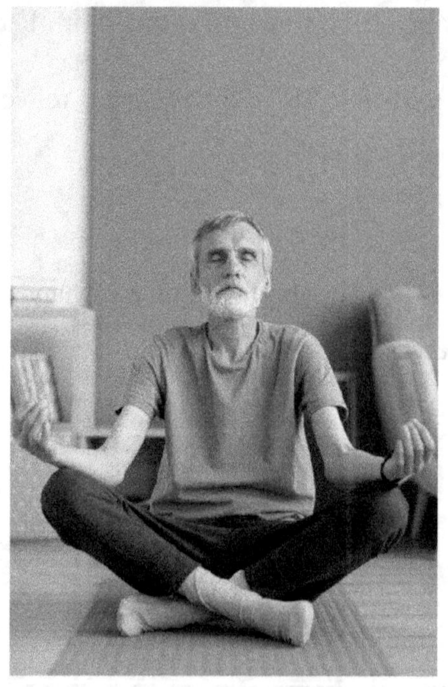

Conclusion

Ultimately, the use of chair exercises by seniors over 50 proves to be a transformational and vital aspect of good aging, rather than just a fad in fitness. There is substantial research, encompassing mental, emotional, and physical domains, demonstrating the several advantages of chair workouts for this population.

Physically, chair exercises provide a low-impact avenue for seniors to enhance their strength, flexibility, and cardiovascular health. The gentle movements cater to the specific needs of aging bodies, reducing the risk of injuries while fostering a gradual yet effective improvement in overall fitness. This adaptability is crucial, allowing individuals to tailor their exercise routine to their unique abilities and gradually progress as their strength and stamina increase.

Chair exercises provide seniors a low-impact way to improve their cardiovascular health, strength, and flexibility. The mild motions address the unique requirements of aging bodies, lowering the chance of injury and encouraging a steady but noticeable increase in general fitness. This flexibility is essential because it enables people to customize their workouts to their own abilities and advance gradually as their strength and endurance grow.

The benefits of chair workouts for cognition go far beyond their physical benefits. Regular physical activity improves cognitive function and lowers the risk of dementia and cognitive decline, according to a body of research. Chair exercises help seniors maintain a holistic approach to their well-being by improving their coordination, balance, and spatial awareness by engaging both their body and mind.

Additionally, chair exercises' psychological advantages are crucial to seniors' general quality of life. Exercise is known to cause the production of endorphins, which naturally elevate mood. Chair exercises offer a social outlet that encourages elders to engage in group activities and fosters a community of support, reducing feelings of isolation and enhancing mental health.

Chair exercises are a popular choice for seniors due to their accessibility and ease, whether they are done at home, in a community center, or even at work. Seniors who incorporate these activities into their everyday routines feel more independent and self-assured as they take charge of their health.

Chair exercises are essentially a comprehensive and empowering way for adults over 50 to age gracefully. Chair exercises are a vital component in the quest of a vigorous and meaningful life during the golden years due to their evidence-based advantages, which include improvements in physical, cognitive, and emotional well-being.

Chair exercises are a compelling and convincing option for enhancing health, happiness, and vitality in this group, especially given their simplicity and effectiveness. This is especially true given our shared goal of improving the quality of life for seniors.

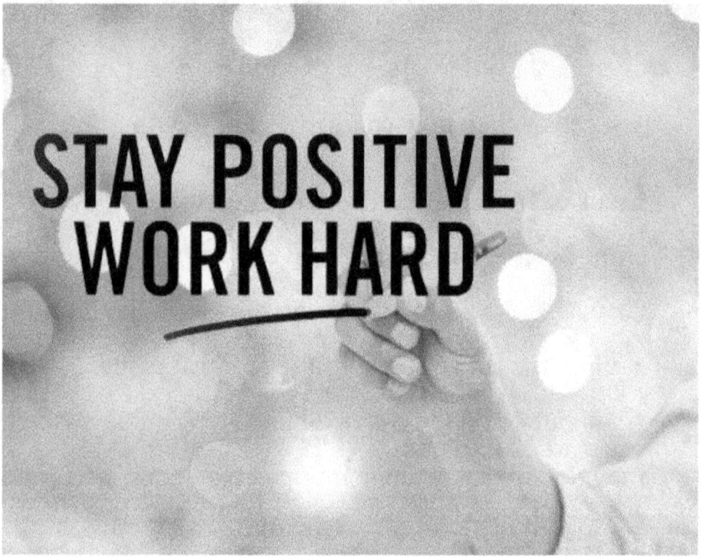

STAY POSITIVE
WORK HARD

PART III: BONUS TIPS FOR SENIORS

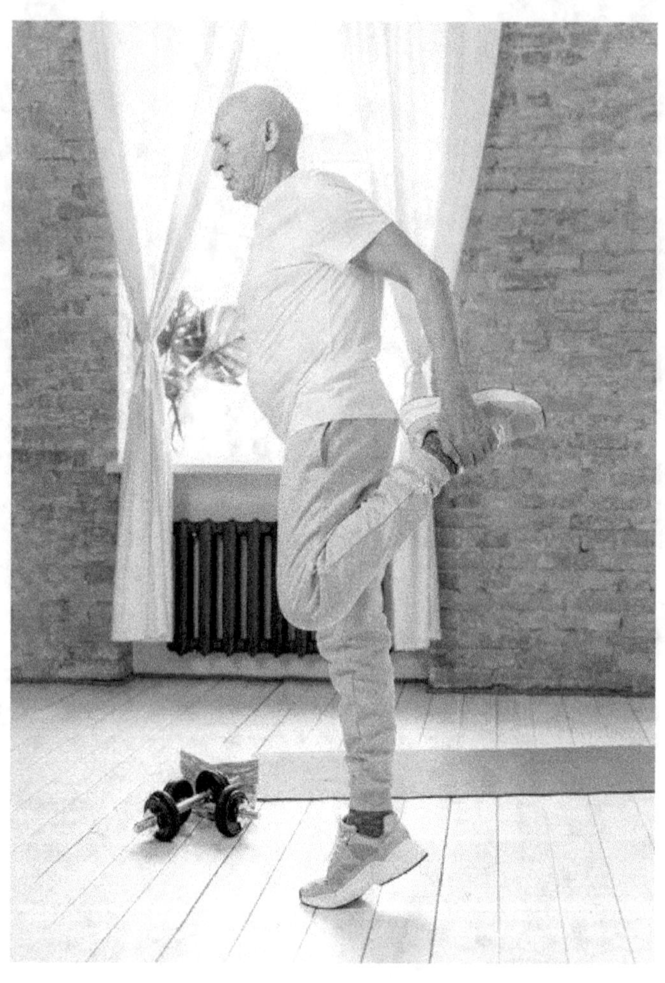

Integrating Wall Pilates and Chair Exercises into Daily Life

For seniors over 50, incorporating chair exercises and wall Pilates into their daily routines is about more than just fitting exercise into a set timetable; it's about incorporating movement into everyday tasks with ease. Without interfering with daily routines, this dual technique combines the stability of a chair with the support of a wall to enhance strength, flexibility, and balance in a comprehensive manner.

1. Wall Stretch in the Morning: Start your day with gentle wall stretches. Lean against the wall while standing with your arms at shoulder height to feel a stretch around your shoulders and chest. This morning exercise produces a good mood for the day.

2. Chair Yoga for Breakfast: Include chair yoga in your morning routine. With the chair's support, you may conduct seated stretches, mild twists, and focused breathing to increase your flexibility and sense of peace before the day starts.

3. Office Chair Pilates Breaks: For those working in an office, Perform chair Pilates during break. To strengthen your core while sitting, try leg lifts, torso twists, or stretches influenced by Pilates.

4. Wall Squats While Cooking: Make spending time in the kitchen a strengthening exercise. Wall squats can be done while you're waiting for water to boil or for a dish to bake. Engage your glutes and thighs as you lower yourself into a sitting position while keeping your back to the wall.

5. Chair Cardio While Watching TV: Transform watching TV into a cardio workout. For arm exercises, leg lifts, and sitting marching, utilize a stable chair. Modestly increase your heart rate to make leisure time into an opportunity for workout.

6. Wall Push-Ups before Bed: Include wall push-ups in your nighttime routine. Stand facing the wall with your hands at shoulder height, then gently perform push-ups. With no additional equipment needed, this workout promotes strength by focusing on the arms and chest.

7. Garden Chair Exercises: Take the chair outside for some gardening activities. Use it for support when performing standing workouts or for seated stretches. Leg raises and calf stretches might benefit from the additional assistance that the wall offers for the legs.

8. Wall Stretch during Phone Conversations: Make the most of your phone calls to stretch your walls. Lean slightly into the stretch while standing up against the wall and extending your arms high. This increases range of motion and also turns inactive moments into active ones.

9. Wall Planks for Lunchtime: Include wall planks in your lunch breaks. Stand and face the wall placing your hands at shoulder height, taking a step back, making a diagonal line with your body. For a low-impact yet high-impact plank variation, engage your core.

10. Chair Relaxation Before Sleep: Use sitting relaxation techniques to unwind before bed. Make a quiet transition to bedtime by using the chair as support for mild stretches and breathing techniques.

Seniors can enjoy the advantages of a thorough training regimen without the commitment of a scheduled gym session by including chair exercises and wall Pilates into their daily lives. This method promotes a conscious and comprehensive relationship between movement and daily activities in addition to improving physical well-being.

28-days workout Challenge for Seniors

Day 1 - 2: Mobility and Foundations

Wall Pilates:

- Wall Squats: stand against the wall with your back, lower yourself into a sitting position and hold for 15 seconds. Perform 10 times.

Chair exercises: Include seated leg raises, ankle circles, and seated torso twists. Perform each for a minute.

Days 3 – 4: Cardiovascular Health

Wall Pilates:

- Wall Marching: Raise your knees to your chest and alternate between your legs for 2 minutes.

Chair Exercise: 3 minutes of vigorous seated marching and seated jumping jacks.

Day 5 – 6: Activation of the Core

Wall Pilates:

- Wall Plank: Put your hands on the wall, stretch your legs back, and hold the position for 30 seconds.

Chair Exercise: Seated leg extensions with abdominal contractions, seated marches with torso twists.

Day 7: Relaxation Day

Both: Wall stretch and chair yoga: Gentle yoga positions focusing deep breathing and emphasizing wall stretching against the wall. Give yourself permission to rest and relax.

Days 8 – 9: Cardio Blast While Seated

Wall Pilates: Wall Sit Leg Lifts: Do leg lifts while maintaining a 2 minutes wall sit position.

Chair Exercise: For 4 minutes, perform vigorous seated marching and arm circles.

Days 10 – 11: Dynamic Arm Workout

Wall Pilates:

- Wall Push-Ups: Take a position arms-length apart from the wall and perform push-ups for 2 minutes.

Chair Exercise: Resistance band workouts, arm lifts, and seated bicep curls.

Day 12 – 13: Seated Cardio Interval

Wall Pilates: Wall Marching Intervals: For 5 minutes, alternate between vigorous wall marching and quick rest intervals

Chair Exercise: Quick sitting marches and jumping jacks in succession.

Day 14: Relaxation Day

Both: Wall stretch and chair yoga: A session focusing on relaxation, deep breathing, and moderate stretches.

Days 15 – 16: Full Body Strength

Wall Pilates:

- Wall Leg Press: Lean against the wall, lift your legs, and apply pressure to the wall for resistance.

Chair Exercise: Push-ups, Seated Squats, and Seated side leg lifts.

Days 17 – 18: Balance and Stability

Wall Pilates:

- Wall Leg Crosses: Stand sideways to the wall, support yourself by crossing one leg over the other.

Chair Exercise: Leg Crosses While Seated, Stability Ball Exercises, and Knee Extensions.

Days 19 – 20: Unwinding and Chair Yoga

Both: Wall Stretch and Chair Yoga: Concentrate on stretching against the wall, breathing techniques, and easy yoga positions.

Days 21 – 22: Endurance Challenge

Wall Pilates: Wall Plank Endurance: Hold a wall plank for increasingly longer periods of time, aim for 3 minutes.

Chair Exercise: Increase the time spent performing arm exercises and fast sitting marching.

Days 23 – 24: Emphasis on Flexibility

Wall Pilates:

Wall Hip Flexor Stretch: Stand and face the wall, lean forward, then notice the stretch in your hip flexors.

Chair Exercise: Wall Stretches for flexibility and Seated Stretches for main muscle groups.

Days 25 – 26: Integration of Whole Body

Wall Pilates:

- Torso Twist with Wall Squat: Do a wall squat while rotating your torso to the left and right.

Chair Exercise: A mix of aerobic, strength, and flexibility movements for a complete workout.

Day 27: Relaxation Day

Both: Wall Stretch and Chair Yoga: Before the last task, try some gentle yoga positions, breathing techniques, and stretching to help you relax.

Day 28: Grand Finale - Full Body Challenge

Both: Wall Combo and Chair: Combine some of the challenge's workouts into a single full-body routine. Celebrate the progress you've accomplished in the last 28 days!

Throughout the challenge, keep your form correct, pay attention to your body, and enjoy the path toward better physical health, mobility, strength, flexibility, and general well-being.

Post-Workout Nutrition Tips for Seniors

When it comes to seniors engaging chair exercise and wall Pilates routines, post-workout nutrition is essential. After exercise, a healthy diet promotes general wellbeing, helps muscles recover, and refills energy reserves. Here's a comprehensive guide to post-workout nutrition tailored for seniors:

1. Rehydration: Seniors should give priority to rehydrating after exercise in order to replenish fluids lost through Sweat. The best option is water, but electrolyte-rich drinks may also be helpful, particularly after a really strenuous workout.

2. Protein Consumption: Protein is necessary for muscular growth and healing. Seniors should try to have a post-workout meal or snack that includes a source of lean protein. Choices consist of:

- **Greek Yogurt:** High in protein and probiotics for muscle health and digestion.

- **Turkey or Chicken:** Lean poultry is a great source of protein.

- **Plant-Based Proteins:** For those following a vegetarian or vegan diet, beans, lentils, and tofu make great substitutes.

3. Carbohydrates to Refuel Energy: After a workout, consuming carbs restores glycogen stores and gives the body the energy it needs to recover. Options include:

- **Whole Grains:** Oats, brown rice, and quinoa are great options.

- **Fruits:** Fruits like apples, bananas, and berries provide natural sugars and vitamins.

- **Sweet Potatoes:** High in fiber and complex carbs.

4. Healthy Fats: Including sources of healthy fats in meals that follow an exercise promotes satiety and overall nutritional balance. Choices consist of:

- **Nuts and Seeds:** Chia seeds, walnuts, and almonds are good sources of fat.

- **Avocado:** A rich source of monounsaturated fats and nutrients.

5. **Antioxidant-Rich Foods:** To counteract oxidative stress from exercise, seniors should consider consuming foods high in antioxidants. Choices consist of:

- **Berries:** Powerhouses of antioxidants include blueberries, strawberries, and raspberries.

- **Leafy Greens:** Vitamins and minerals are found in spinach, kale, and Swiss chard.

6. **Protein Smoothies:** A protein smoothie is a handy choice for seniors, particularly those who have trouble chewing or have limited appetite.

Blend:

- Plant-based protein powder or Greek yogurt

- Mixed berries

- Banana

- Water or milk (dairy or plant-based)

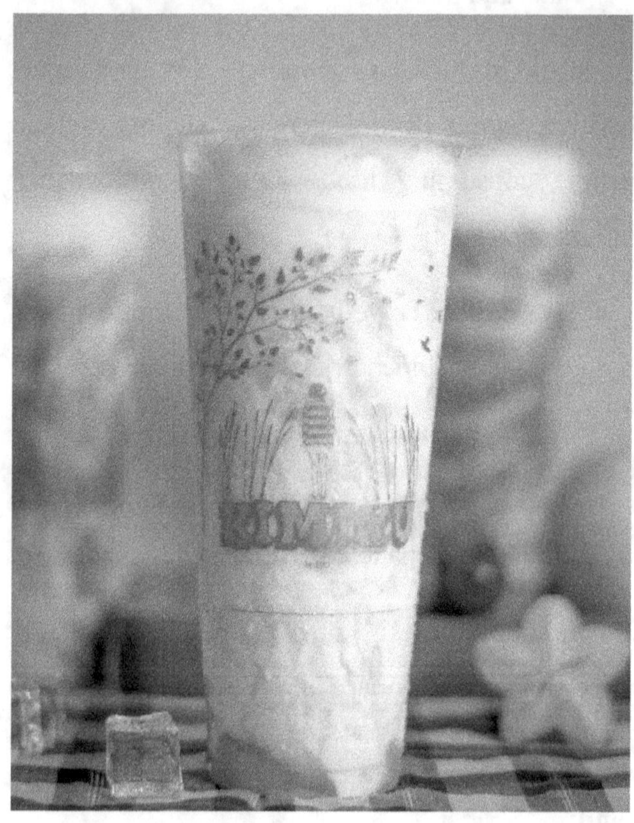

7. When to Eat after a Workout: To optimize the advantages of nutrient absorption, seniors should ideally eat a post-workout meal or snack within 30 minutes to an hour after exercise. However it's important to be flexible, and eating a delayed post-workout meal is preferable to skipping it completely.

8. Customized Nutrition Plans: Individual nutritional needs differ, so seniors should consider consulting a licensed dietitian or nutritionist for individualized guidance based on their health conditions, food preferences, and level of exercise.

Key Points to Consider:

- **Hydration Matters:** Make sure you're getting enough fluids intake to help your recovery and avoid dehydration.

- **Listen to Your Body:** To decide the right portion sizes, pay attention to your body's signals of hunger and fullness.

- Regular Nutrients Intake: Rather than depending exclusively on post-workout nourishment, seniors should concentrate on sustaining a regular nutritional intake throughout the day.

By incorporating these post-workout nutrition guidelines, seniors engaging in wall Pilates and chair exercises can improve their recovery, support muscle health, and maximize the advantage of their exercise routine. For long-term wellbeing, it's critical to customize dietary decisions to each person's requirements and tastes.

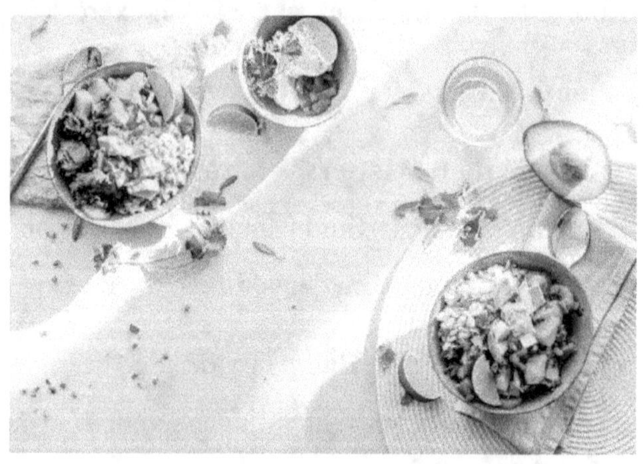

Staying Motivated and Engaged

Embarking on a journey of wall Pilates and chair exercises is admirable for seniors, and maintaining motivation is key to long-term success. Here are a few tips to keep the enthusiasm alive:

1. Appreciate Small Wins: Honor and appreciate every accomplishment, no matter how minor. Every step you take forward is evidence of your commitment and development.

2. Variety is the Spice of Life: Make your workouts interesting by varying them up. Try out new chair exercises, experiment with different Pilates routines, or add good rhythm to your sessions.

3. Create Achievable and reasonable Goals: Create attainable and reasonable goals. This might be learning a new Pilates pose, lengthening the time of your workouts, or boosting your flexibility. Achieving small, manageable goals makes you feel accomplished.

4. Socialize through Exercise: Participate in online courses or group activities with pals. Interacting with others while working out fosters a sense of community and adds a fun factor.

5. Pay Attention to Your Body: Pay attention to your body's signals. Adjust the workout to your comfort level if it seems too difficult. Enjoying the process without undue stress is crucial.

6. Establish a Routine: Make an exercise schedule that you stick to. Exercise becomes an indisputable part of your day when you set aside a specific time for it, which promotes discipline.

7. Maintain Your Curiosity: Approach your exercises with an open mind and a desire to learn. This kind of thinking keeps things interesting and makes it easier to find new routines that you enjoy doing.

8. Reward Yourself: After hitting a fitness benchmark, treat yourself to a modest treat. It may be time spent alone with a nice book, a favorite nutritious food, or a soothing bath.

9. Evaluate Your Progress: Consistently consider your progress. Making progress visible to yourself is a great way to stay motivated and to push yourself farther.

10. Embrace the Pleasure: Above all, take pleasure in the process. Exercise is a chance to enjoy the movement, energy, and vitality it gives to your life in addition to its benefits to your physical health.

Recall that maintaining motivation is an individual process. Seniors can design a regimen that is fun and sustainable and improves their general well-being by adding variation, setting realistic goals, and finding joy in the movement.

"Each move you
made is a step
toward vitality.
You've got this!"